MY QUOTABLE PATIENTS

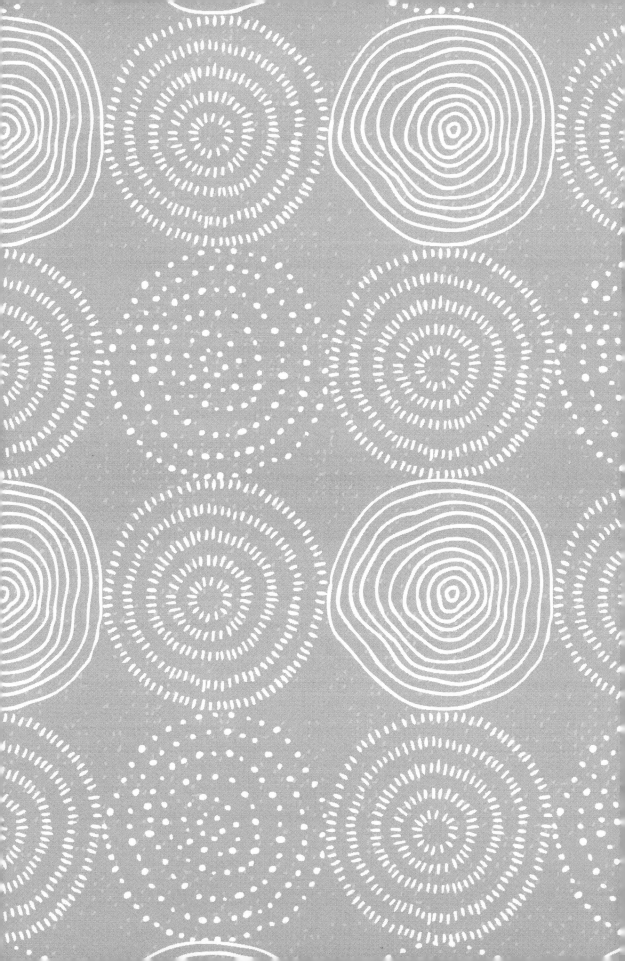

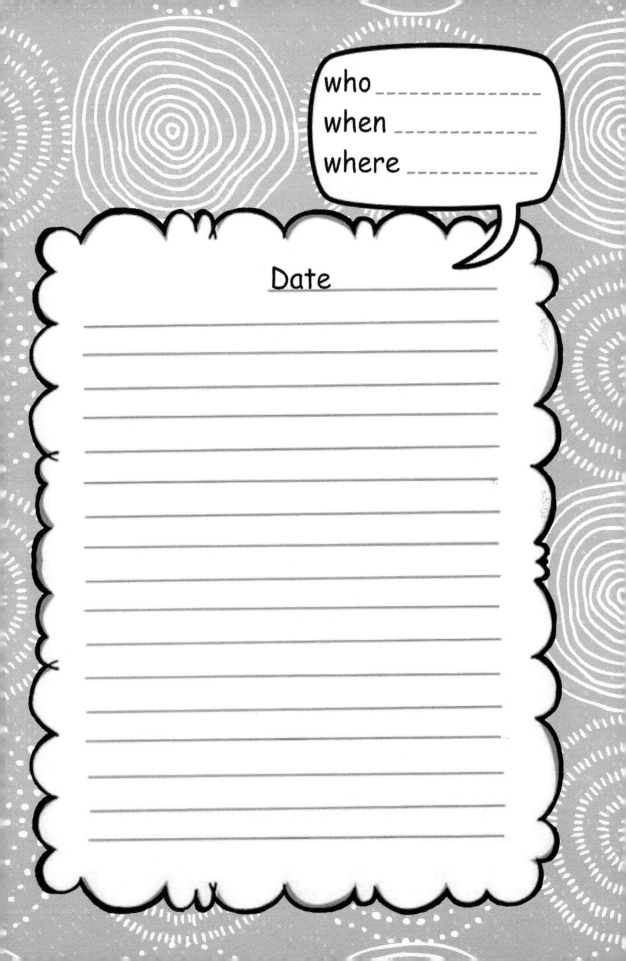

who _____

when _____

where _____

Date _____

who _____

when _____

where _____

Date _____

who _____

when _____

where _____

Date _____

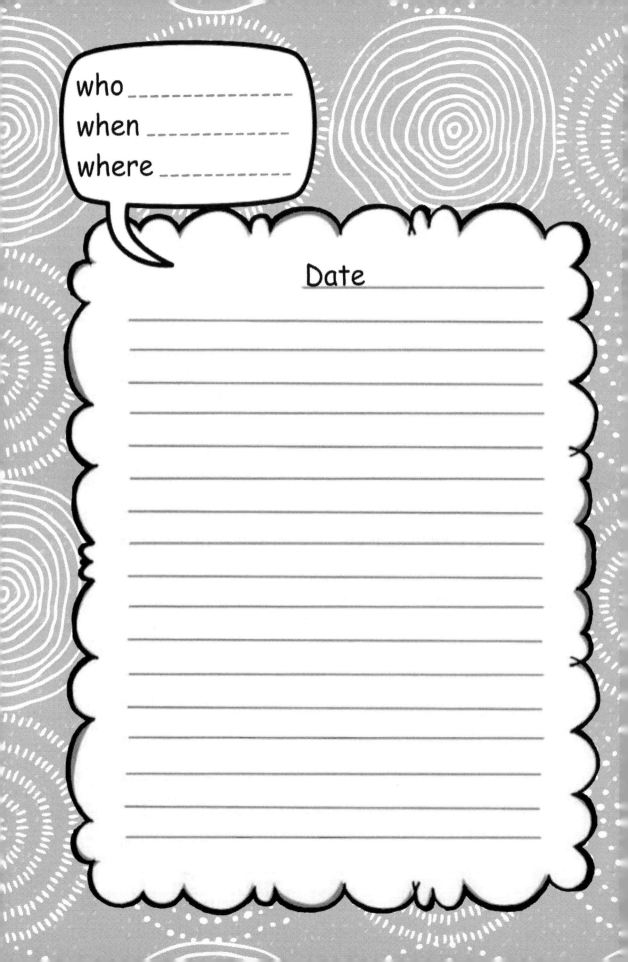

who _____

when _____

where _____

Date _____

who _____

when _____

where _____

Date _____

who _____
when _____
where _____

Date _____

who _____
when _____
where _____

Date _____

_____
_____
_____
_____
_____
_____
_____
_____
_____
_____
_____
_____
_____
_____

who _____
when _____
where _____

Date _____

who _____

when _____

where _____

Date _____

_____
_____
_____
_____
_____
_____
_____
_____
_____
_____
_____
_____
_____
_____
_____
_____

who ____________

when ____________

where ____________

Date ____________

who _____
when _____
where _____

Date _____
_____
_____
_____
_____
_____
_____
_____
_____
_____
_____
_____
_____
_____

who _ _ _ _ _ _ _ _ _ _ _

when _ _ _ _ _ _ _ _ _

where _ _ _ _ _ _ _ _

Date _____

who _____

when _____

where _____

Date _____

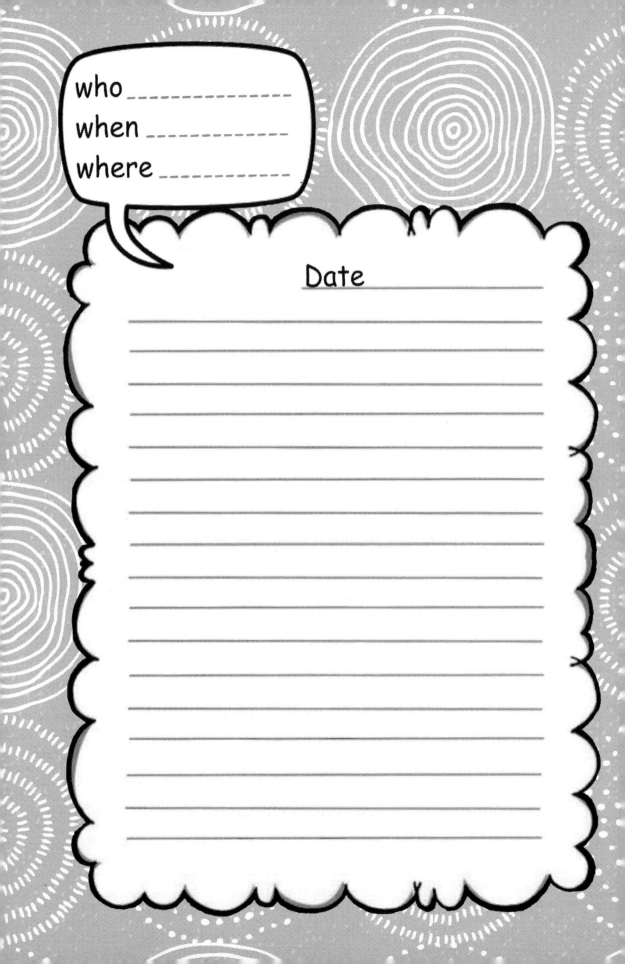

who _____

when _____

where _____

Date _____

who _____

when _____

where _____

Date _____

who _____

when _____

where _____

Date _____

who _____

when _____

where _____

Date _____

_____
_____
_____
_____
_____
_____
_____
_____
_____
_____
_____
_____
_____
_____
_____
_____
_____

who _____

when _____

where _____

Date _____

_____
_____
_____
_____
_____
_____
_____
_____
_____
_____
_____
_____
_____

who _____

when _____

where _____

Date _____

_____
_____
_____
_____
_____
_____
_____
_____
_____
_____
_____
_____
_____

who ______________
when ____________
where ____________

Date ______________________

who _____

when _____

where _____

Date _____

who _____

when _____

where _____

Date _____

who _____

when _____

where _____

Date _____

who _____

when _____

where _____

Date _____

who _____

when _____

where _____

Date _____

who _____
when _____
where _____

Date _____

who _____

when _____

where _____

Date _____

who _ _ _ _ _ _ _ _ _ _ _ _ _ _
when _ _ _ _ _ _ _ _ _ _ _ _
where _ _ _ _ _ _ _ _ _ _ _

Date _____

who _____

when _____

where _____

Date _____

_____
_____
_____
_____
_____
_____
_____
_____
_____
_____
_____
_____
_____
_____

who _____

when _____

where _____

<u>Date</u> _____

who _____
when _____
where _____

Date _____

_____
_____
_____
_____
_____
_____
_____
_____
_____
_____
_____
_____
_____
_____
_____

who _____

when _____

where _____

Date _____

who _____

when _____

where _____

Date _____

who ______________

when ______________

where ______________

Date ______________

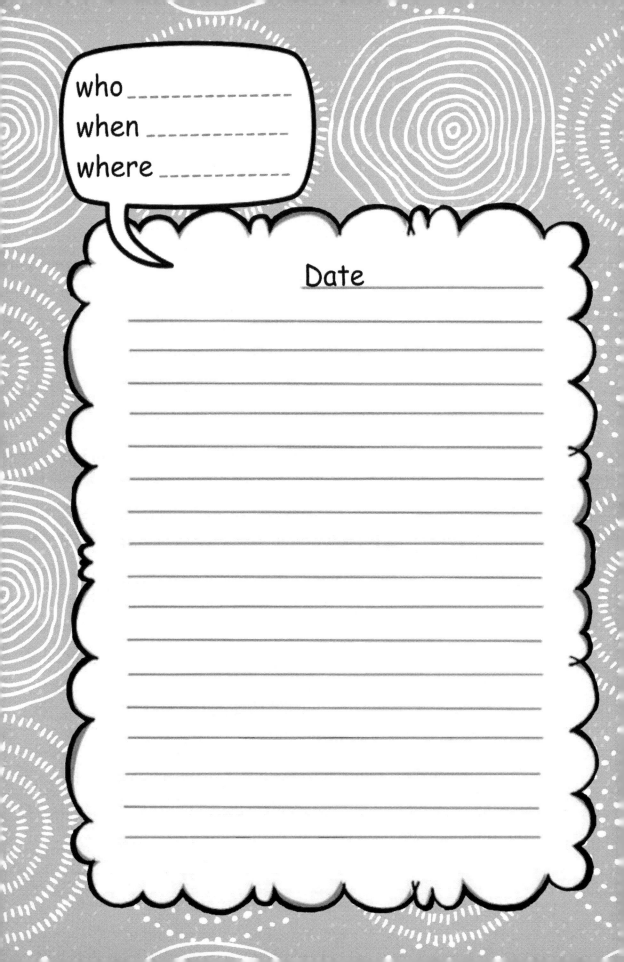

who _____

when _____

where _____

Date _____

_____
_____
_____
_____
_____
_____
_____
_____
_____
_____
_____
_____
_____
_____
_____
_____
_____
_____

who _____

when _____

where _____

Date _____

who _____

when _____

where _____

Date _____

who ______________
when ____________
where ___________

Date ______________________

who _____

when _____

where _____

Date _____

who _____
when _____
where _____

Date _____

who _____

when _____

where _____

Date _____

_____
_____
_____
_____
_____
_____
_____
_____
_____
_____
_____
_____
_____
_____
_____

who ____________

when ____________

where ____________

Date ____________

who _____

when _____

where _____

Date _____

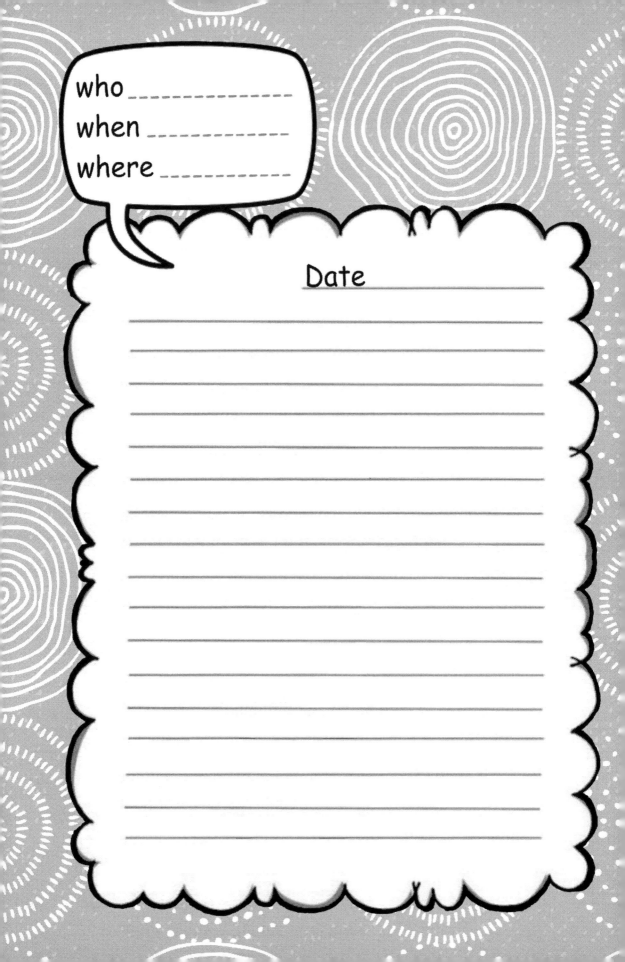

who _____

when _____

where _____

Date _____

who _____

when _____

where _____

Date _____

_____
_____
_____
_____
_____
_____
_____
_____
_____
_____
_____
_____
_____
_____
_____
_____
_____
_____
_____

who _____

when _____

where _____

Date _____

who _____
when _____
where _____

Date _____
_____
_____
_____
_____
_____
_____
_____
_____
_____
_____
_____
_____
_____
_____
_____
_____
_____

who _____

when _____

where _____

Date _____

who _____

when _____

where _____

Date _____

_____
_____
_____
_____
_____
_____
_____
_____
_____
_____
_____
_____
_____
_____
_____
_____
_____
_____

who ______________

when ____________

where ___________

Date ____________________

who _ _ _ _ _ _ _ _ _ _ _ _ _

when _ _ _ _ _ _ _ _ _ _ _

where _ _ _ _ _ _ _ _ _ _

Date _____

who _____
when _____
where _____

Date _____

who _____

when _____

where _____

Date _____

_____
_____
_____
_____
_____
_____
_____
_____
_____
_____
_____
_____
_____
_____
_____
_____

who _____

when _____

where _____

Date _____

who _____

when _____

where _____

Date _____

who _____
when _____
where _____

Date _____

who _____

when _____

where _____

Date _____

who _____

when _____

where _____

Date _____

_____
_____
_____
_____
_____
_____
_____
_____
_____
_____
_____
_____
_____
_____

who _____
when _____
where _____

Date _____

who ______________

when ______________

where ______________

Date ______________

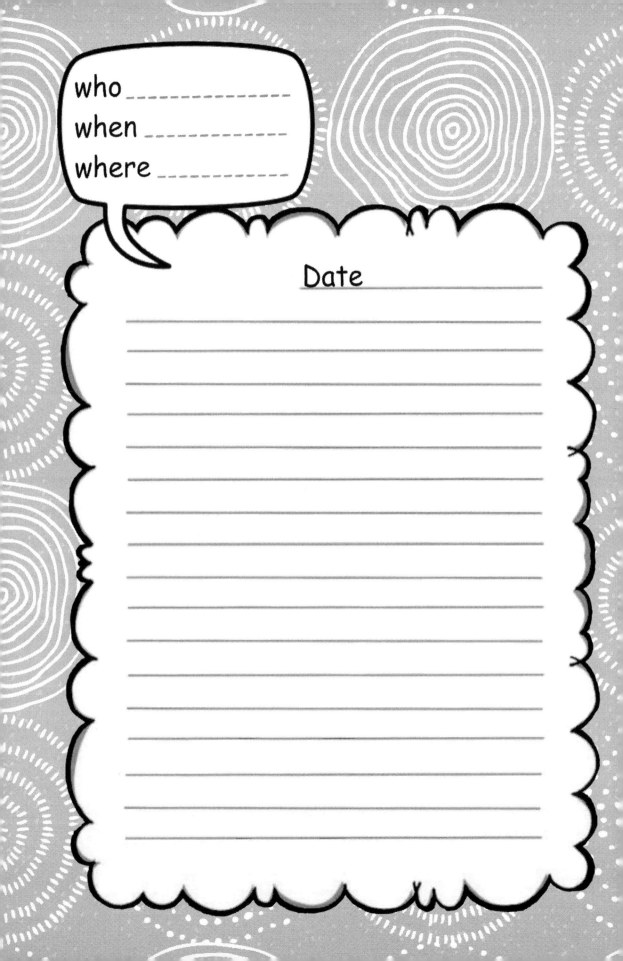

who _____
when _____
where _____

Date _____

who ____________

when ____________

where ____________

Date ____________

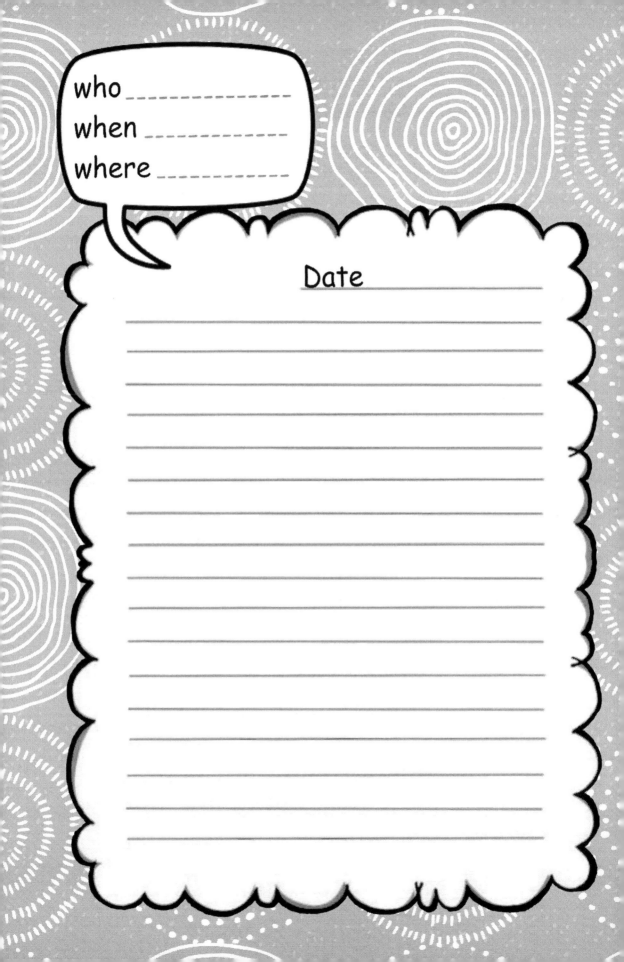

who _____

when _____

where _____

Date _____

who _____

when _____

where _____

Date _____

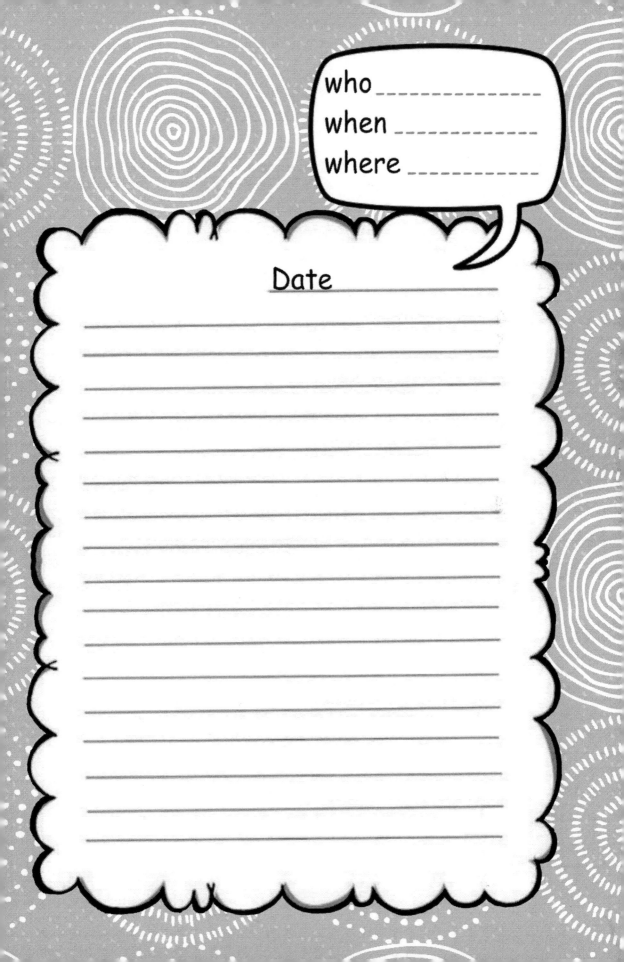

who _____

when _____

where _____

Date _____

who _____

when _____

where _____

Date _____

who _____

when _____

where _____

Date _____

who _____
when _____
where _____

Date _____

who ______________

when ______________

where ______________

Date ______________

who _____

when _____

where _____

Date _____

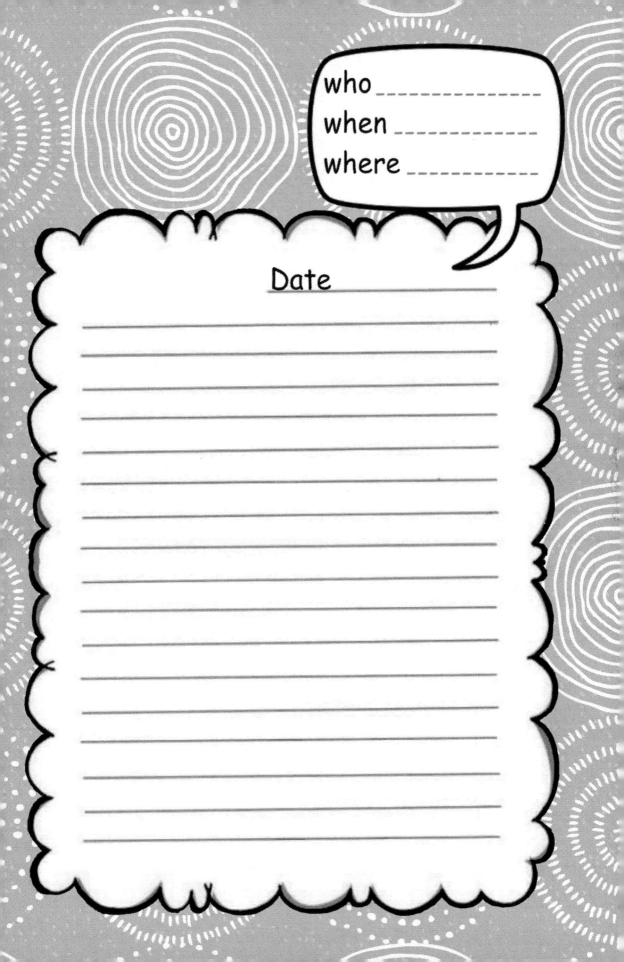

who _____

when _____

where _____

Date _____

who _____

when _____

where _____

Date _____

who _____

when _____

where _____

Date _____

_____
_____
_____
_____
_____
_____
_____
_____
_____
_____
_____
_____
_____
_____
_____
_____

who _ _ _ _ _ _ _ _ _ _
when _ _ _ _ _ _ _ _ _
where _ _ _ _ _ _ _ _ _

Date _____

who _____

when _____

where _____

Date _____

_____
_____
_____
_____
_____
_____
_____
_____
_____
_____
_____
_____
_____
_____
_____

who _____

when _____

where _____

Date _____

who _____

when _____

where _____

Date _____

who _____

when _____

where _____

Date _____

who ______________

when ____________

where ___________

Date ________________________

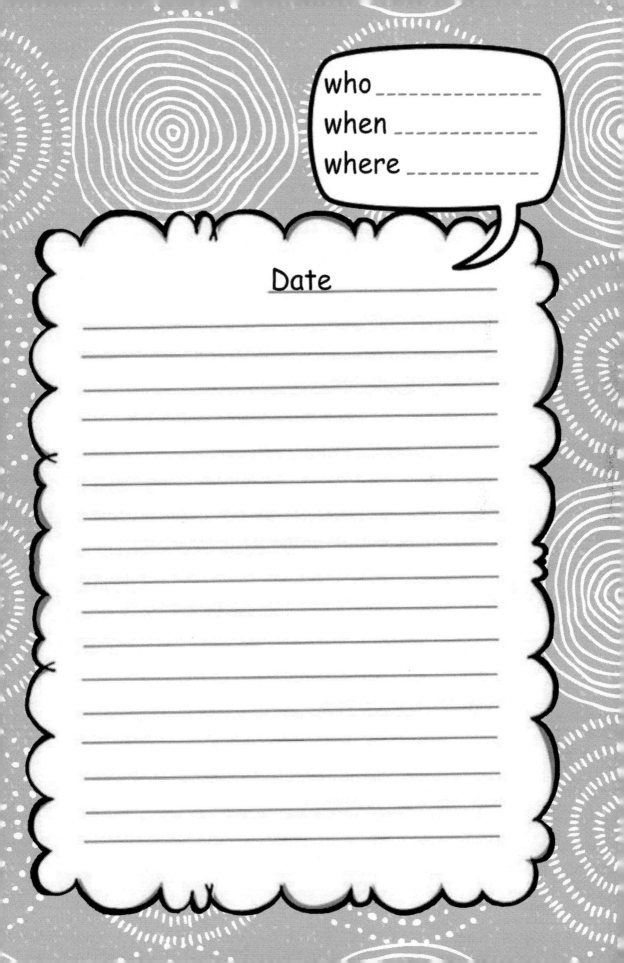

who _____
when _____
where _____

Date _____

who _____
when _____
where _____

Date _____

who _____
when _____
where _____

Date _____

_____
_____
_____
_____
_____
_____
_____
_____
_____
_____
_____
_____
_____
_____

who _____
when _____
where _____

Date _____

who _____

when _____

where _____

Date _____

who _____

when _____

where _____

Date _____

_____

_____

_____

_____

_____

_____

_____

_____

_____

_____

_____

_____

_____

who _____

when _____

where _____

Date _____

who _____

when _____

where _____

Date _____

_____

_____

_____

_____

_____

_____

_____

_____

_____

_____

_____

_____

_____

_____

_____

_____

_____

who

when

where

Date

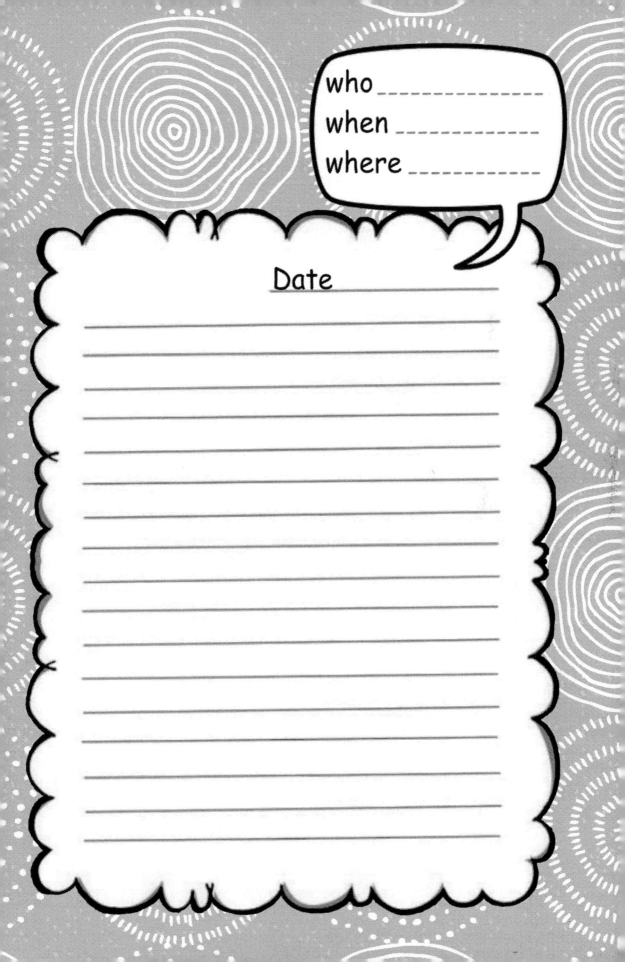

who _____
when _____
where _____

Date _____

who _____
when _____
where _____

Date _____

who _____

when _____

where _____

Date _____

_____

_____

_____

_____

_____

_____

_____

_____

_____

_____

_____

_____

_____

_____

_____

_____

who _____

when _____

where _____

Date _____

who _____

when _____

where _____

Date _____

who _____

when _____

where _____

Date _____

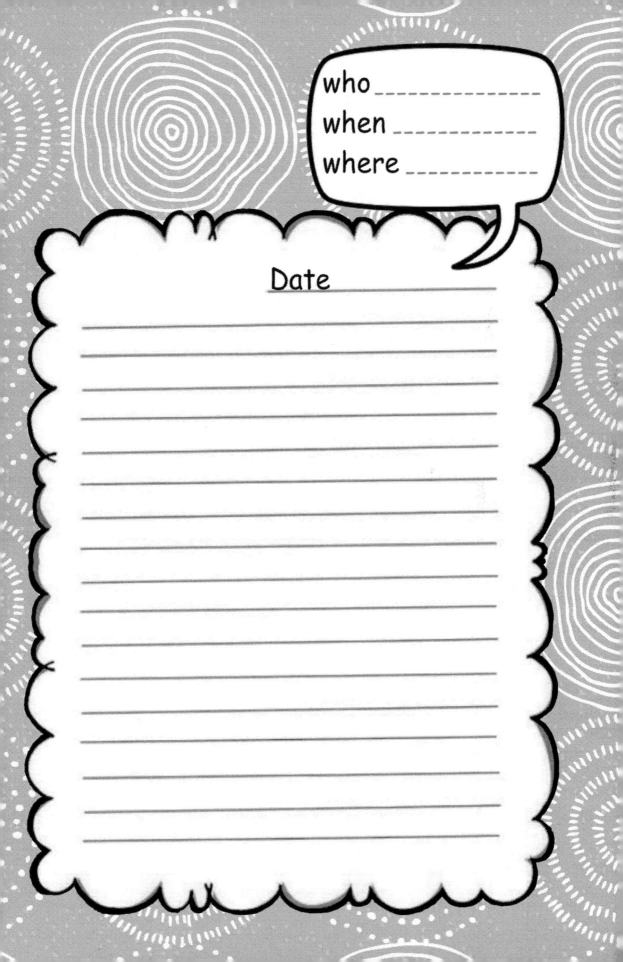

who _____
when _____
where _____

Date _____

who _____

when _____

where _____

Date _____

_____
_____
_____
_____
_____
_____
_____
_____
_____
_____
_____
_____
_____
_____
_____

who _____

when _____

where _____

Date _____

who _____

when _____

where _____

Date _____

_____

_____

_____

_____

_____

_____

_____

_____

_____

_____

_____

_____

_____

_____

who _____
when _____
where _____

Date _____
_____
_____
_____
_____
_____
_____
_____
_____
_____
_____
_____
_____
_____
_____
_____
_____
_____
_____

who _____

when _____

where _____

Date _____

who _____

when _____

where _____

Date _____

who _____

when _____

where _____

Date _____

who _____

when _____

where _____

Date _____

who _____

when _____

where _____

Date _____

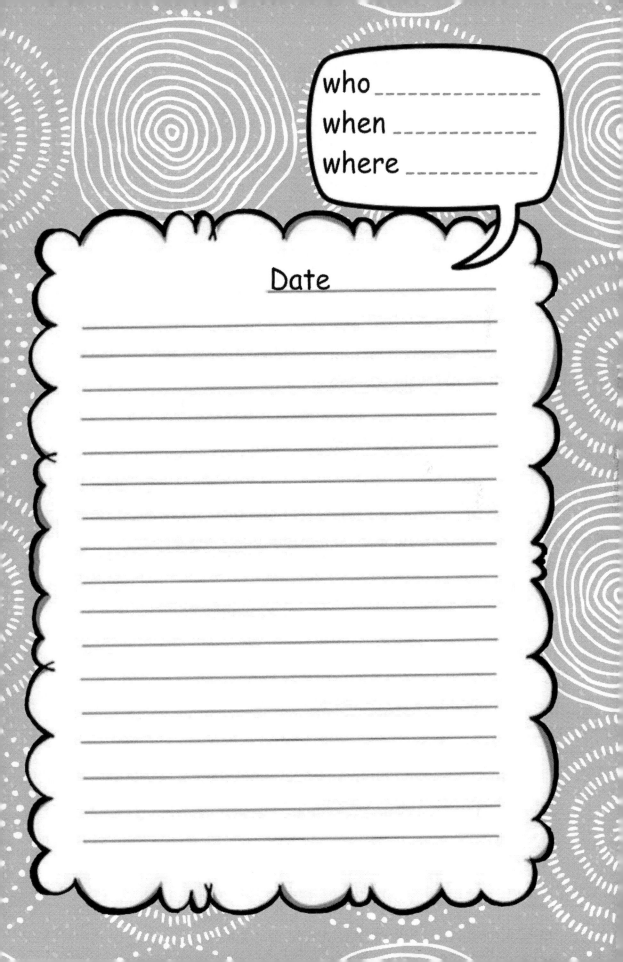

who _ _ _ _ _ _ _ _ _ _ _ _ _

when _ _ _ _ _ _ _ _ _ _ _

where _ _ _ _ _ _ _ _ _ _

Date _____

who _____
when _____
where _____

Date _____

Made in the USA
Coppell, TX
08 June 2021